Make Aromatherapy Work

How Sweet It Is To Use Aromatherapy Daily: Hidden Secrets

By: Helga Shaffer

9781680322446

PUBLISHERS NOTES

Disclaimer – Speedy Publishing LLC

This publication is intended to provide helpful and informative material. It is not intended to diagnose, treat, cure, or prevent any health problem or condition, nor is intended to replace the advice of a physician. No action should be taken solely on the contents of this book. Always consult your physician or qualified health-care professional on any matters regarding your health and before adopting any suggestions in this book or drawing inferences from it.

The author and publisher specifically disclaim all responsibility for any liability, loss or risk, personal or otherwise, which is incurred as a consequence, directly or indirectly, from the use or application of any contents of this book.

Any and all product names referenced within this book are the trademarks of their respective owners. None of these owners have sponsored, authorized, endorsed, or approved this book.

Always read all information provided by the manufacturers' product labels before using their products. The author and publisher are not responsible for claims made by manufacturers.

This book was originally printed before 2014. This is an adapted reprint by Speedy Publishing LLC with newly updated content designed to help readers with much more accurate and timely information and data.

Speedy Publishing LLC

40 E Main Street, Newark, Delaware, 19711

Contact Us: 1-888-248-4521

Website: http://www.speedypublishing.co

REPRINTED Paperback Edition: ISBN: 9781680322446

Manufactured in the United States of America

DEDICATION

I dedicate this book to my family. I am always grateful to have you.

TABLE OF CONTENTS

CHAPTER 1- ANCIENT USE OF AROMATHERAPY

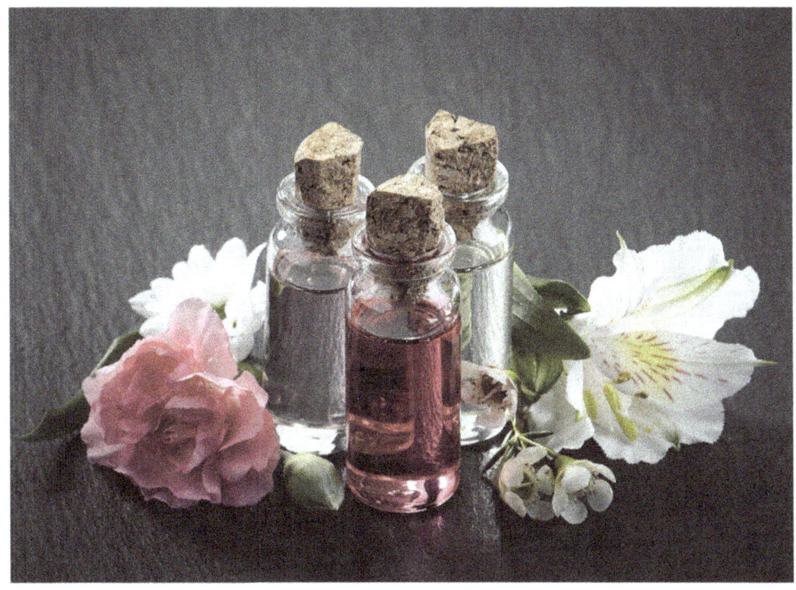

You may have heard of Aromatherapy but you probably have no idea what it is or how it can change your life. Perhaps you've seen ads for aromatherapy massage or even purchased what you thought were aromatherapy candles in the store. Most likely, you don't understand much about aromatherapy or the wonderful healing powers possessed by true aromatherapy.

Aromatherapy is an ancient Eastern art that has been practiced for thousands of years. Although it is hardly anything "new" it sometimes takes a little bit of time for people in the West to discover such things such as natural healing, especially when it is not in the best interest of the very powerful medical and pharmaceutical communities.

Those of us who live in the West have an entirely different mindset than those in the East. In the West, when someone gets ill, they go to the doctor who more often than not, prescribes medication to treat or cure the ailment. The medication is produced in a laboratory and contains synthetic chemicals. Pharmaceuticals are big business and doctors are often courted by sales people from the companies to prescribe their product.

Go to a doctor in the West for a bit of anxiety and they will prescribe anti depressants such as Zoloft. Chances are your doctor will have a prescription pad in his or her hand when they walk into the room. Zoloft is among the many different anti depressant medications that are relatively new on the market and lumped under SSRIs. The long term side effects of these drugs are not known, although they will most likely cause liver damage after long usage.

No doctor it the West will prescribe any alternative treatment, such as aromatherapy. Some might tell you to exercise and take vitamins to combat anxiety, but most won't even do that. The medical community dances on the strings held by the pharmaceutical companies and the name of the game in pharmaceuticals is to give people synthetic drugs that are addictive and costly so that they can make money.

One hundred years ago, heroin was used as a cough medicine for children. Cocaine was put into Coca Cola and arsenic was considered "good for the complexion." Perhaps, one hundred years from now, our descendants will be talking about how people were prescribed lethal substances to "cure" them from various ailments.

Aromatherapy is not a "new drug" just off the market. Aromatherapy is all natural. It consists of using essential oils in various ways to promote healing. Essential oils are derived from all natural products such as plants, trees, fruit, etc. There are over 100 essential oils commonly used today and they are used to treat a variety of different maladies, just as they have been for thousands of years.

Bunk? Most doctors will tell you that aromatherapy is a crock, even though the essential oils have been used for such a long time and have been imitated in synthetic products produced by laboratories. It is not in the best interest of the medical community for you to stay healthy. They want you to keep coming back to get those pills for minor ailments.

The pharmaceutical companies are very powerful in the West. They fear aromatherapy and will denounce it. They would rather have you buy their chemicals for $2 a pill than use something from nature that costs hardly anything at all.

But when you look at aromatherapy with logic and understand where how it works, it makes perfect sense. Everything we need to survive is found in nature. We have food, water, air - all from nature. Take a look at the way a trees and plants give off oxygen and grow with carbon dioxide. See how human beings do the opposite. Everything in nature is very well balanced.

It makes sense that nature would also provide us with cures for any ailments our bodies or minds may suffer. While many in the medical community feel that depression and anxiety are a result of a chemical imbalance in the brain, why can't those chemicals be balanced with the use of natural products? Why do we always rush first towards synthetics?

In the West, we are of a mindset to turn away from nature, rather than embrace it. Things are different in the East. This is why the life span of those in Eastern countries is longer than those in the West, despite the fact that they do not visit the doctor as often as we do and many of them smoke. Rates of cancer in the West are much higher than in the East as well. Why?

The practice of aromatherapy involves embracing nature at its best. Using essential oils in your everyday life, not only to heal, but to maintain good health in both body and spirit. Essential oils are pure and natural and most have a pleasant scent. When you incorporate aromatherapy into your daily life, you can change your life for the better.

In the next few chapters, you can learn all about how to use aromatherapy in variety of different ways. You will also learn some simple recipes to make with essential oils as well as where to purchase essential oils and the different types of products you can make. You'll even learn how you can use aromatherapy in your own business, or even start a business using this Eastern healing art.

Whether you want to stay healthy or cure a minor ailment, aromatherapy can help. Using this timeless art can really make quite an improvement in your everyday life.

Aromatherapy dates back to ancient cultures more than 5,000 years. In continents like Africa, certain plants were eaten by warriors before going into battle. Most of the time, the healing powers of the plants or barks were observed after animals had consumed the foliage or fruit. The animal's behavior was observed and humans found that they, too, could get the same effect.

Horny goat weed is an example of a plant that has been used for ages to increase fertility in men. Despite the funny sounding name this natural derivative was discovered after horned goats were found getting very frisky and having high energy levels after consuming the plant. It has been used for centuries as a product to treat impotence.

While herbal remedies have been used in most countries for thousands of years as a way to stay healthy and combat illness, the concept of aromatherapy, which is using the scented oils derived from the plants to cure and heal, got its roots, so to speak, in the far East.

Lavender is a pleasant scented flowering plant that is grown all over the world although it grew naturally in warm climates. Lavender is grown widely today for the oils that are used for everything from sweetening certain dishes to being used as an antiseptic.

The essential oils derived from this plant can be used to treat headaches, as a cure for insomnia and to promote relaxation. Lavender is one of the few essential oils that is safe to use directly on the skin and can also be consumed. Essential oils are not made for oral ingestion, but lavender buds are sold as a tea in some health food stores. Lavender has been used for thousands of years to treat everything from insect bites to anxiety.

Because it has an antiseptic quality, lavender was also used to disinfect floors in hospitals. Today, most disinfectants are chemically produced and toxic to both those who use them as well as to the environment.

It was the Ancient Chinese who first discovered the many healing powers of the various essential oils and gave it a name. Herbal medicine is still practiced in the far East today and many people from the west travel to countries such as Thailand and Singapore to find relief in natural herbal remedies and treatments.

Thousands of years ago, villagers would visit someone in the village who knew all about the different herbal remedies and would treat them accordingly.

Most people also had some knowledge of the different plants that grew around them and how they could be used to benefit their lives. Today, however, most people have no idea how to even use simple herbs to add flavor to a recipe, let alone use them for healing.

Most people in the west pay little attention to the plants and nature around them or any healing powers that those plants may contain. This is gradually beginning to change. Many people today, thanks to the internet, are beginning to understand a little about herbal remedies and aromatherapy.

As the ancient Chinese used scents to heal, the concept was delivered to the ancient Egyptians who created mixtures of the scents and made perfumes. The scents were not only used to heal illness, but also as an aphrodisiac.

The ancient Egyptians incorporated aromatherapy into their daily rituals and were the first perfumers.   In ancient Egyptian, it was once a requirement that everyone perfumed themselves at least once a week and people often took three baths a day in perfumed water.

Sandalwood is used in incense for its pleasant scent and the Ancient Egyptian women would use the oils from Sandalwood in their hair for the scent. Other scents were also discovered that were both pleasant and healing.

Throughout centuries, different cultures used the essential oils derived from nature for a variety of products and healing ointments. Herbal remedies were also very popular treatments for ailments until the discovery of penicillin. Penicillin was derived from mold, also a natural substance, and was used to treat bacterial ailments and infections.

Today, penicillin remedies are known as antibiotics and are produced in laboratories with synthetic materials.

The history of Aromatherapy may date back to ancient times, but it was widely accepted in all cultures until chemicals began replacing the natural essential oils. Today, aromatherapy is considered alternative medicine that many people are finding a better choice than a dependency on synthetic chemicals.

Chapter 2- Experience the Soothing Effects of Aromatherapy

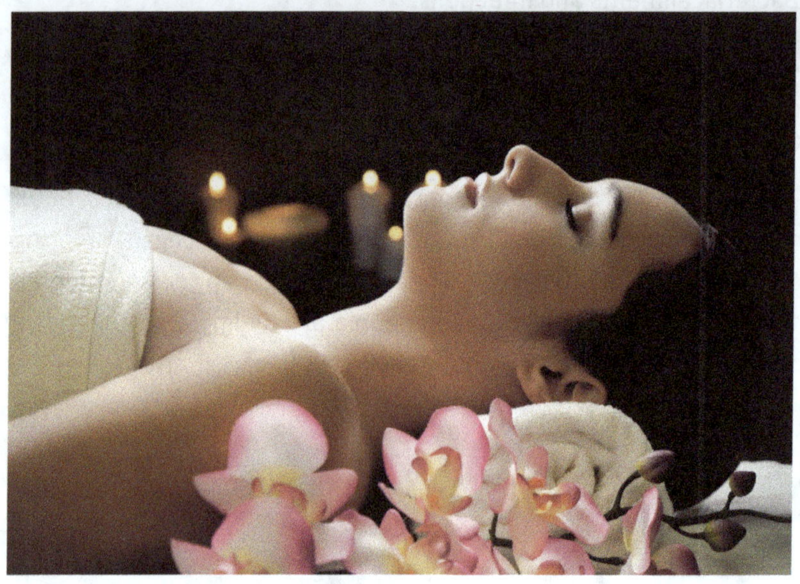

Aromatherapy massage oils are derived from a blend of essential oils. In order for the aromatherapy to work properly, the essential oils have to be 100 percent pure. Do not be fooled by synthetic products that claim to be "aromatherapy." True aromatherapy massage oils are100 percent natural and contain only pure essential oils.

We all know how soothing massage therapy can be. Just the massage alone, in most cases, is enough to calm and relax us. When aromatherapy is incorporated into the massage, it doubles the effect.

As the essential oils are absorbed into your skin, they find their way into your blood stream and begin to soothe and heal. Aromatherapy massage oils can be used for a variety of purposes. The three most common uses for an aromatherapy massage are:

- Relaxation

- Sexual stimulation

- Pain relief

Depending upon which essential oils are blended as well as the massage techniques will determine the outcome.

Although many people seek to get an aromatherapy massage by a licensed massage therapist for relaxation, this is something that you can do at home. You can actually make your own aromatherapy massage oil if you know which type of blends to use and how to use them.

Before you begin making aromatherapy massage oils in your home, it is very important that you observe the following rule:

Never use essential oils directly on the skin. Essential oils are very concentrated and should always be diluted with a carrier oil when being used in massage therapy. There are exceptions, such as lavender and vanilla, but as a rule of thumb, dilute essential oils with a carrier oil before using directly on the skin.

That caveat aside, you can easily make your own massage oil at home and begin incorporating aromatherapy into your daily life.

You will want to make sure that the essential oil that is used is 100 percent pure essential oils. Again, most products that claim to be aromatherapy are not. The one way you can be certain of getting true aromatherapy massage oil is to actually make it yourself.

There are a variety of different outlets where you can purchase pure essential oils. Some of them are very inexpensive, such as lavender, while others, such as sandalwood, can be costly. Check out the glossary at the end of this book for a list of online retailers that sell pure essential oils.

In addition to the essential oils, you will also need a carrier oil. Because the essential oils are so highly concentrated, you only need about eight drops of the oils to one ounce of the carrier oil. Popular choices for carrier oils include:

- Apricot kernel oil

- Sweet almond oil

- Common vegetable oil

Yes, common vegetable oil can be used as an effective as well as very inexpensive, carrier oil for an aromatherapy massage oil.

Storing massage oil should be done in dark colored bottles with a seal. Most places that sell aromatherapy products online, such as essential oils, also sell bottles and other supplies. It is important for you to store the aromatherapy massage oil in a dark glass in a cool, dark place as the oil can lose its effectiveness if exposed to light.

The aromatherapy massage oil can be directly mixed in the bottle where it will be stored. Simply measure an ounce of the carrier oil, pour it into the bottle and then add about eight drops of your blend of essential oils. If the essential oil does not come with a glass dropper, you need to purchase one of these products. A glass eyedropper is necessary when working with essential oils as a plastic dropper will react with the oil.

The glass dropper that you use should not have a rubber top. Rubber can also react with the essential oils. Again, most places that sell essential oils online also sell the proper supplies that you need to use the oils.

Once you have added the two oils together, seal the bottle and roll it around in your hands gently to mix the oils thoroughly. You should make sure that you do this before each and every use. Do not shake the bottle vigorously, but gently roll it to mix the oils.

You can pour a little bit of the oil into a bowl and heat it in the microwave for a few seconds prior to use. You must make sure that it is not too hot before applying the blend to the skin. Massage oils feel better on the skin when used warm. No one like cold oil drizzled on them as it can be a bit unpleasant.

Prior to using aromatherapy massage oils, do a test patch on the skin. Some people have very sensitive skin that can have an allergic reaction to the oils. Make sure you test it out prior to putting it all over your body or that of someone else to make sure it does not cause an allergic reaction.

The massage oil can be used on the torso, arms and legs as well as the head and neck area. Avoid the eyes, ears, mouth and genital areas as well as any areas of inflammation or broken skin. The oils will begin to work upon being absorbed into the skin and entering the blood stream.

While you may think of massage as something that you need to have done by another person, or do to another person, you can also treat yourself with aromatherapy massage oils. For example, you can rub your temples with a lavender massage oil to ease a headache. You can also rub your feet and hands with massage oil.

There are various types of massage techniques that you can learn, although true massage therapy is actually studied and is a healing art all unto itself. For an amateur, however, learning to rub certain areas of the body is not difficult. The back is a primary source of tension and an aromatherapy back rub can do wonders to relieve stress.

As the cells that promote healing within our immune system are found in our upper digestive system, rubbing the front torso with healing aromatherapy oil can also be beneficial. For a sensual massage, you will want to rub the legs, buttocks and chest area.

Mild anxiety

Following are three popular recipes that are commonly used for relaxation, sexual stimulation and pain relief:

Aromatherapy Massage Recipe For Relaxation

1 ounce of carrier oil 5 drops of lavender

3 drops of sandalwood

You can also substitute Rose or Mandarin for Sandalwood in the above recipe. By reading the glossary of essential oils contained in the book, you can learn which oils can do what.

For relaxation, make sure that you also set the mood. Light some candles and play some soothing music. Massage your partner with warmed massage oils beginning at the base of the neck and working your way down his or her back. Rub shoulders and muscles throughout the back and allow the magic of the healing oils to go to work.

Aromatherapy Massage Recipe For Sexual Stimulation

1   ounce of carrier oil 6 drops of jasmine

2   drops of bergamot

Jasmine is a safe and effective way to promote confidence and stimulation. For a loving treat, use an aromatherapy massage on your partner to help him or her relax and enjoy lovemaking. Speak soothingly and lovingly to your partner as you use this tried and true blend.

Aromatherapy Massage Recipe For Pain Relief

1   ounce carrier oil 4 drops chamomile 4 drops tea tree

A deep tissue massage, or a Swedish massage, is one way to alleviate pain that is caused by physical activity. You can use this recipe blend to sooth aching feet by rubbing firmly with your thumbs into the souls of your feet as well as the heel.

This aromatherapy massage treatment can also be used on the body and is especially good at relieving joint pain for arthritis sufferers.

There are many other uses for aromatherapy massage. Once you become familiar with the concept of aromatherapy and the different uses for essential oils, you can make your own blends and treat a variety of minor ailments such as:

Insomnia

Menstrual cramps

Bruises

Mild depression

Stress

Memory improvement

Anger relief

Aromatherapy massage is one of the most effective alternative healing methods used today. Although it has been used for centuries, the demand for massage therapy has doubled in the past decade. It looks as if many people have discovered the benefits of healing through aromatherapy massage treatment and is on their way to feeling good naturally.

Chapter 3- Aromatherapy for Sensitive Skin

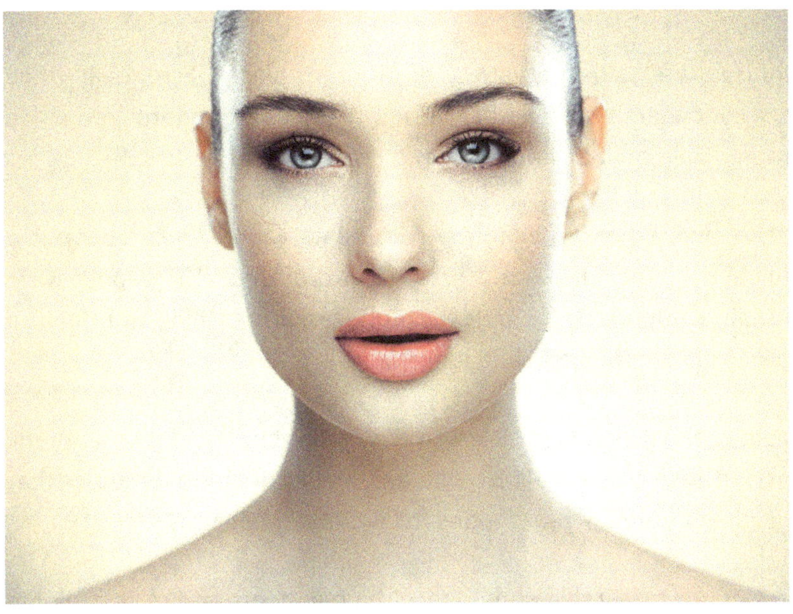

Many people who have sensitive skin may think that they cannot enjoy the healing benefits of this art because of a sensitive skin condition. Wrong! If you have sensitive skin, you can still enjoy aromatherapy as it was truly meant to be enjoyed - just by scent.

We talked about using aromatherapy in perfumes as an aphrodisiac. Not only does the perfume cause the person who is using it to become aroused, but it can cause others who catch the scent o also become aroused. In this way, another individual is responding to aromatherapy through scent.

You have probably noticed different oils in the store that claim to give the benefits of aromatherapy. Most of these oils are synthetic and do little more than cosmetically cover up odors in your home. While having your home smell nice is a good bonus, it is not main use of aromatherapy.

When inhaled into the lungs, essential oils cause the same reaction in an individual as they will when applied to the skin. This means that you can just enjoy heating the oils in an infuser and breathing them in to cure what ails you.

Infusers are sold in a variety of different places. Essentially, they are containers that can heat oil and send it wafting throughout the room. They can be heated either by candle or by electric.

Years ago, when ill, people would heat "vapors" in a pot, put a towel over their head and breathe in the fume. The vapors were usually camphor. This would promote easier breathing and clear up congestion in the head and lungs.

Today, people who get sick rush to the drugstore and buy synthetic pills to ease congestion. No one ever thinks of home remedies that had been used for generations to cure minor ailments.

This is not to say that someone with pneumonia or a serious illness should ignore medical advice and try to cure themselves using essential oils. That would be irresponsible and foolish. However, someone who has a stuffy nose does not have to rush off and take pills. There are other avenues that are more natural and even more effective.

The same goes for depression. Chronic depression or depression that lasts for more than two weeks is a serious illness and should be treated by a physician. Someone who is suffering from anxiety attacks that are causing them to miss work or hyperventilate should seek medical help. Someone who has a broken leg or infected finger should go to a doctor.

That being said, someone who is a little bit upset because they broke up with a boyfriend or girlfriend or may just be suffering from the blues does not need to rush to the doctor to get on SSRIs. Someone who is a little anxious about taking an exam for school does not need tranquilizers and someone who is sore because they work out a lot should not resort to addictive pain medication or even abuse over the counter pain pills.

There is another way to treat minor ailments and conditions and that way is aromatherapy.

Furthermore, there is nothing to say that using aromatherapy in conjunction with medications cannot do wonders. Many people are enjoying the benefits derived from this alternative medicine that has been effective for thousands of years.

When using aromatherapy as a mood enhancer in an infuser, you do not need to dilute the oils. You can use any oils that you want, or a combination of oils, to set the mood. Here are some ways you can use aromatherapy in a variety of different infusers:

Aromatherapy Mood Enhancer Recipe

5 drops of orange 5 drops of jasmine

Sure that you do not use the scents that are sold in the craft stores as they are usually not true essential oils but synthetic scents. Follow the directions on the box to make the candles.

Put them into an infuser that is either plugs into an electric socket or is heated by a candle and allow the scent to permeate the room.

Aromatherapy Romantic Mood Enhancer

This is simple - put a couple of drops of patchouli, jasmine or Ylang Ylang on the light bulb in your room. The light bulb can be used to heat the oil and will spread the scent in the room. All of these oils are potent aphrodisiacs.

Aromatherapy Relaxing Infusion

Get an electric infuser that is used to heat potpourri oil and put it in your room on your dresser. Add the following:

10 drops chamomile

2 drops vanilla

2 drops lavender

This will allow you to really relax as the scent takes over the room. Scent has quite a bit to do with how we feel. The scent sends a signal to our brain and releases endorphins. You can actually put yourself in a better mood by scent, which is the basic concept of aromatherapy.

When we talk about aromatherapy today, we are discussing the use of essential oils to promote healing. However, the scent is a vital aspect to the healing powers involved in this alternative medicine. Even when you are using essential oils in a topical way, you are still breathing in the scent and getting the full effect of the true treatment.

You do not only have to use aromatherapy to heal. You can just use the essential oils as a way to make your home smell nice for all who visit. Because they are so concentrated, essential oils work well in homes where there is smoking or pets.

Other ways to use essential oils as an infusion method is to make your own candles. Candle making is not difficult. You simply need to melt wax and add color and scent. The color is actually optional. You have to put the melted wax into a container or mold with a wick so that it can be lit.

Making your own candles using essential oil is one of the best ways to continue to get the same effect of the oil. To make your own candles, go to a craft store such as Hobby Lobby or Michael's and pick up a large brick of wax along with some wicks and wick holders. Wick holders are little metal fragments that keep the wick affixed in the mold. You can keep the wick straight by tying it around a pencil and laying the pencil across the top of the container.

You will have to heat the wax in a pot on the stove or, preferably, over a double boiler. The wax will seem like it is taking forever to melt, but once it starts, it melts very quickly so be prepared to remove it from the stove as soon as it melts all the way. You will see that the white chunk of wax is now clear.

You can then add about 10 drops of your essential oil to about every cup of wax. There are also dyes you can purchase to color the candles.

Blend it with a spoon and pour the wax into jars or a mold. Allow the candles to set in room temperature over night. Make sure that the wicks are standing up straight before the wax sets. A candle without a wick is useless.

When you light the wick, it will begin to melt the wax and the scent will be given off into the room. You can light the candle any time you want and begin to get the effects of the essential oil immediately.

If you have never before made candles, get candles making kit. Candle making with essential oils not only promotes healing, but can be a fun thing to do for the entire family. Young people in particular like to make candles. One of the first crafts that kids make in school is the old "milk carton candle." Your children and you will not only enjoy making the candles, but also be able to benefit from the pleasant and healing scent that they emit.

Incense

Incense has been used for thousands of years, mostly in religious ceremonies. Ancient Egyptians used incense to heal as did the ancient Chinese. Today, incense is still a vital part of certain religious ceremonies, particularly in the Catholic and Orthodox religion.

People also use incense for a variety of different reasons, in most cases, to mask certain odors. Incense can also be incorporated into you aromatherapy lifestyle if you use pure essential oil powders to make your own incense.

Today's incense is usually cones or sticks and is made, like everything else, with synthetics. Sure, they have a pleasant fragrance, but you are not getting the same benefits as you can get with incense made from pure and natural products.

If you decide to make your own incense, realize that it takes a bit of time to get it right. The incense cones that you create will be hand crafted, as will the sticks. They may not look as uniform as those you buy in the store, but they will have more healing powers than anything made with synthetics.

To make incense at home, you will need powders as well as essential oils. The essential oils should be the same as the powder so that it complements the product; You also need to purchase Makko powder, which can be purchased at the same places where you buy the essential oils and powders. '

Sandalwood is one of the oldest and most pleasant aromas. To make sandalwood incense at home, use about half sandalwood powder to half Makko powder. Put both in a bowl and add about four drops of sandalwood essential oil. You then need to mix it together to make dough.

Once you have the thoroughly blended, you can roll it into long sticks. This is probably the easiest way to make the incense. There is actually spaghetti makers that you can use to perform this process that will make the sticks come out more even; however, you should not use the same machine to make spaghetti. If you have an old spaghetti maker around, you might give it a try.

Just like spaghetti, you will want to make sure the sticks dry out on waxed paper before they are ready to use. It takes a couple of days for them to dry completely. You want to make sure to cut them so that they are compatible with your incense burner. Incense burners that burn sticks are usually long, wooden instruments or boxes.

If you really want to get creative, you can also make cones out of the dough. The cones will probably not look like those in the store, but they will be just as effective when lit. You do need to make sure that any homemade incense is completely dried out before using.

Sandalwood is a woodsy fragrance that is very rich. It has been used in the past to treat everything from stress to bronchitis. Because of the pleasant fragrance, we also illustrated how sandalwood oils can be used to scent your hair simply by sprinkling a few drops on your brush and brushing your hair as usual.

Although aromatherapy incense may not look as good as the incense you purchase in the store, it can be a lot of fun to make and is really very simple. Once you have made an enjoyed your own incense made out of all natural essential oils, you will not want to go back to using store bought oils again.

Make sure that you have a proper incense burner to light the incense and never leave it burning unattended.

Chapter 4- Aromatherapy for Bath and Beauty Essentials

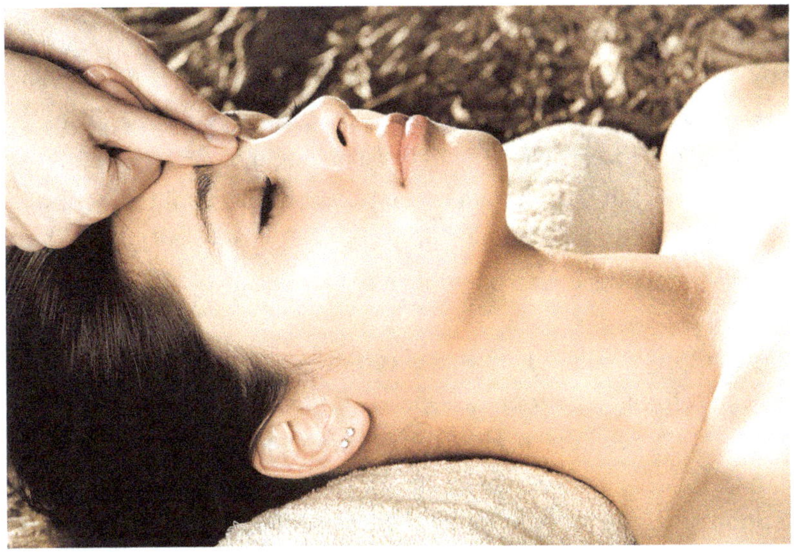

Now that you have a concept of how to use aromatherapy as a massage treatment, you can probably imagine using these precious essential oils in the bath. Aromatherapy bath products include bath salts and oils.

Aromatherapy bath oils can be used to treat you in the same manner as massage oils. The concept is basically the same - you take a warm and relaxing bath with water that contains about a quarter of a cup of aromatherapy bath oil. The oils go to work when they penetrate the skin.

Again you will want to test the bath oil to make sure that it does not cause an allergic reaction. If you want a truly relaxing bath, use lavender or vanilla as both of them are among the safest and most mild oils to use. Rose also makes good bath oil.

Making your own aromatherapy bath oil is simple and economical. Yes, essential oils can be costly, but as you only need a few drops, it can last quite a long time. Again, you will want to use carrier oil, but vegetable oil is very inexpensive. You will also want to use the glass eye dropper and the dark colored bottles that you can purchase online.

You can make enough bath oil to last for a few baths by doubling the recipe and adding two ounces of carrier oil to 20 drops of essential oil. The ratio for the bath oil is roughly the same as it is for massage oil, but you can add a couple more drops of the essential oil as it is also being diluted into water. On the average, add 10 drops of essential oils to one ounce of carrier oil.

The bath oil should be store in a cool, dark place. Most likely, you will want to put it in your bathroom cabinets. As is the case with all products that you make, keep the bottles away from children.

A popular recipe for relaxing bath oil is as follows:

Aromatherapy Relaxing Bath Oil Recipe

2   ounces of carrier oil 12 drops of lavender

6   drops of rose

2   drops of tea tree

Be sure that you blend the oils properly as you would for massage oils and only use about a quarter of a cup of oil in the bath. Lavender rose and tea tree are all very pleasant and will provide you with soothing relief in the bath.

If you are having menstrual cramps or any sort of stomach pain, you can also use the following:

Aromatherapy Pain Relief Bath Oil Recipe

2 ounces of carrier oil 10 drops of rose

4   drops of peppermint

6   drops of chamomile

Soaking in a warm tub is one way to relieve stomach cramps caused either by stress or your menstrual cycle.

The bath oil will have a shelf life of a year. Once you have experimented with taking an aromatherapy bath, you will probably toss away all of the synthetic chemicals you have been using in your bath water and begin enjoying a true, natural healing bath.

If you want to make bath salts to put into the bath, you can also do the same. You will need Epson salts or Dead sea salts. Both are available online and Epson salts are very inexpensive and available at your local drug store.

The ratio for the bath salts is three cups of salts, one tablespoon of carrier oil and about 20 drops of essential oil. These are mixed in a bowl with a spoon or a fork until very well mixed. Then you can put them in a jar with a tight fitting lid. Store them in a dark place. You can put about a half a cup of the salts into the tub under warm running water and wait for them to dissolve when you step in.

Bath salts are very popular because they store easier and you don't have to worry about spilling.

You can use the above recipes for bath oils for bath salts by just making the proper substations.

If you want to color the bath oils to make them look pretty, you can use exotic salts such as Hawaiian Red Sea salt which has a natural salmon color. You can even mix these with the Epson salts. Commercial producers of bath salts usually use a mica powder to color the salts that are also used in color cosmetics.

You are better off, however, leaving the bath salts in their natural state so as not to cause any skin irritation. Do not use vegetable oil food dyes to color the salts as they can turn the skin that color in the bath and will take a few washes before rinsing out of the skin.

Another recipe for bath salts that is good for general relaxation and to help you settle for sleep is as follows:

Calming Bath Salts Aromatherapy Recipe

3 cups of Epson salts 1 tablespoon carrier oil 10 drops chamomile

5 drops lavender

4 drops tea tree

1 drop lemon

You will enjoy taking a bath in aromatherapy bath salts that can cure aching joints and bones, ease tension, relieve cramps and sooth you prior to going to bed. Once you begin making bath oils and bath salts, you will most likely give them as gifts to friends who can also enjoy their helpful benefits.

Beauty Products

Once you discover the world of essential oils and aromatherapy, there is no end to what you can do. You will most likely want to incorporate this ancient healing art into every aspect of your life, including your beauty and hygiene routine.

The great thing about using essential oils is that they are 100 percent natural. No synthetic ingredients. This not only makes them safer for you, but also safer for the environment. You can learn to use aromatherapy in much of your beauty routine.

One way to have instant, shining hair that is lightly scented is to sprinkle a couple of drops of sandalwood on your hairbrush. Brush your hair as usual and the scent will remain. Sandalwood is one of the more expensive of the essential oils but has a pleasant, woody scent. You can also substitute rose for sandalwood if you want to go a more inexpensive route.

Perfumery is a science. Making your own perfume with essential oils, however, can be fun. Today's perfumes are made with synthetic copies of essential oils as real oils would be too expensive to use in the mass production of perfume.

Most perfumes on the market today are diluted with alcohol and water. You can also use oil to dilute your perfume, although using alcohol will make them last longer. When making perfumes, you will want to experiment with a variety of different fragrances. Most perfumes fall into one of the five categories:

Woodsy

Floral

Oriental

Spicy

It takes a bit of experimenting with essential oils to get the scent that you want. Most perfumes are usually a blend of three different "notes."

They contain one or more from each of the above categories. There is a base note, a mid note and a top note. The top note is the first to evaporate on your skin. It is also the first impression that you have of the fragrance. The mid note stays on a little bit more and the base note is what will remain on your skin for hours.

The base note will react with your skin to form a scent of its own. This is why no two perfumes smell exactly alike on any two people. It is also the reason why you should test out a perfume for about a half an hour by putting a dab on your wrist, doing your shopping and then taking a sniff to see if you still like the scent.

The nice thing about using aromatherapy perfumes that you make yourself is that the essential oils can actually help heal anything troubling you, or even give you energy, while also giving you a pleasant scent. Because they are made with synthetics, regular perfumes cannot boast of this power.

You will want to store your perfumes similar to how you store your massage oils - in dark colored glass bottles with tight fitting lids. There is quite a difference when it comes to ratios when making perfumes, however, and they are meant to be used sparingly. You will only be diluting the perfume with one tablespoon of carrier oil or alcohol to about 30 drops of essential oils. As you can see, the ratio between essential oils and either carrier oil or alcohol is almost equal.

As when using any essential oils, do a brief test on your skin before using. Then you are ready to blend.

For floral notes, you can use rose, lavender or geranium. For woodsy notes, you can use sandalwood, myrrh or frankincense. For Oriental notes, use Mandarin, Jasmine or Ylang Ylang. Spicy notes can be ginger, neroli, or nutmeg. The citrus notes are orange, lemon, lime and grapefruit.

It takes a bit of experimenting when making perfumes at home. Perfumery is an art unto itself and takes years to practice. Perfumers today still practice this art and make scents that fail. It is all a matter of personal taste and seeing what blends well with what.

One nice perfume recipe that you can use is very simple and combines woodsy with Oriental:

Basic Perfume Recipe - Oriental

1 tablespoon of carrier oil 15 drops of sandalwood 5 drops of jasmine

4 drops of Ylang Ylang

Watch out - this is quite a romantic perfume! Perfumes were often used as aphrodisiacs and to attract a mate. This one is no different. It has a unique scent a pleasant base note, but again, perfume scents are very subjective. Be sure to experiment a little before you decide to open up your own perfumery.

You just need a little bit of this perfume on your wrists and behind your ears to carry the scent with you through the day. Because the essential oils are so concentrated in this blend, you do not want to use too much.

There is an old saying that your perfume should not walk in the room before you do. You want people to remember pleasant scent, not be overpowered with fragrance.

In addition to being a pleasant perfume, the above aromatherapy fragrance also works to promote energy as well as putting you in a mood for romance. Both jasmine and Ylang Ylang are powerful aphrodisiacs, so only use this one with caution and when you are in the mood for amour.

By the above example, you can probably figure out what type of perfumes to use to relax you as well. The benefits of using aromatherapy in your own perfumes are the following:

Completely natural products and non toxic

Have healing powers as well as a pleasant fragrance

You can have a scent that no one else has (don't underestimate this one - there are people who pay plenty to create their own scent at perfumeries in Paris).

Much less expensive in the long run.

The disadvantages? You have to play around with scents for a little bit before you hit on what you like. Make sure that you write each ratio of every essential oil used in a particular scent as nothing can be more frustrating than actually coming up with the fragrance of your dreams and then not remembering how you ended up making it.

Acne Treatment

Acne is a scourge that mostly affects younger people. It is usually caused by an imbalance in hormones and has nothing to do with eating chocolate, contrary to popular myth.

The treatment of acne generally entails going to a physician and getting medication such as tetracycline, or using over the counter ointments.

You can use certain essential oils that have been used for centuries to heal cuts and infections, to treat acne breakouts.

When using aromatherapy to treat acne, you will want to make sure that you use a light carrier oil. There are light vegetable oils on the market today which work better than a heavy oil. The essential oils that promote healing for acne include lavender, which is pretty much a cure-all for everything, bergamot and tea tree.

Because it is one of the few essential oils that are safe to use directly on your skin, you can use lavender alone and put a drop on the affected area. Or you can use this recipe:

Acne Treatment Aromatherapy Recipe

1 ounce of carrier oil 15 drops lavender

4 drops bergamot

2 drops lemon

Like tetracycline, an oral drug often used to treat acne, bergamot is also photo toxic. This means that exposure to the sun after use can have adverse affects. If you have ever taken tetracycline to combat acne, you know that you need to stay out of the sun while on the medication. The good thing about using bergamot, however, is that you need only stay out of the sun for about 12 hours after use.

This means that you can put the treatment on at night before you go to bed and then rinse off in the morning before going out. It is a lot easier to use than tetracycline and just as effective.

Treating acne also involve healing from the inside. In addition to creating a topical ointment to combat acne, you can eliminate stress by using aromatherapy. There are some indications that some acne breakouts are caused by stress. Use aromatherapy as a means to relax yourself, either in the bath or as a massage treatment.

Chapter 5- Great Concept of Aromatherapy

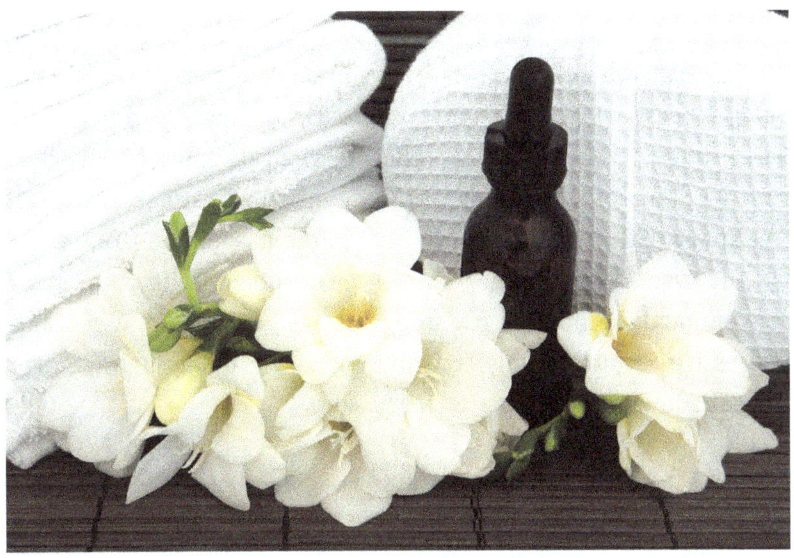

The importance of understanding a particular topic, idea, or element is often overlooked in this busy world of today. To make matters worse it is often difficult to find the time to really extensively explore particular topics. However with the use of various modern tools, this task can be not only fun but very informative too.

Most people today understand aromatherapy as just another indulgent exercise the privileged few enjoy. However upon taking the time to delve deeper, one is likely to find a whole new prospect relating to the very diverse uses of aromatherapy.

Aromatherapy can be explored as an alternative to more invasive methods of treatments. Originating long before medical science made discoveries and break-through; aromatherapy has had many success stories to back its many wondrous attributes. The concept of using aromatherapy to treat wounds and burns first came about when a scientist badly burned his hand while conducting an experiment and later it was used again successfully, as an antiseptic to treat the wounded soldiers during world war two.

Being the basis of natural materials, aromatherapy is less dangerous a method to choose from, when deciding on the best suited treatment for various illnesses. In theory aromatherapy is a treatment that may or may not help in the prevention of diseases by the use of essential oils. When coupled with the more conventional methods of treatments it has been found to produce impressive results, mainly contributing as a calming ingredient to the equation.

Aromatherapy can have a positive impact on the limbic system through the olfactory system. It has also been known to have direct pharmacologic effects. There have been studies done to prove the connection between the direct impacts of use between aromatherapy coupled with other scientific methods, however to date no conclusive data has been forth coming.

Sometimes divided into three distinctive areas of uses, aromatherapy has proven an effective solution to many problems. Aerial diffusion falls in the category for environmental fragrance or disinfection.

Direct inhalation is encouraged to arrest various respiratory problems like respiratory disinfection, congestion, tightness in the chest cavity and many others. Topical applications are mainly for relaxing purposes such as massages, baths, compresses and therapeutic skin care treatments.

Theoretically aromatherapy has been encouraged to be looked upon as an alternative to more invasive type of treatments. Besides being much more pleasant as a treatment option it can sometimes even be touted as a prevention element to certain diseases.

At worst it can play a major role in relaxing the general state of an individual and perhaps contribute in some way to the more successful percentage of recovery when combined with other more scientifically accepted methods of treatment.

Today there are many avenues of treatment to explore before embarking on a particular type suitable for the individual. However it must always be noted that before making a choice, one must always try to be as well informed as possible.

Considering Aromatherapy

Some consider aromatherapy as a new age alternative style of treatment, while yet others know of its origins that date back a long while.

Indulging in aromatherapy is a choice that should only be made after understanding the various aspects of this field. This is most important when choosing aromatherapy as an alternative to medical treatments when trying to arrest, cure or prevent diseases.

What To Think About

The general perception of aromatherapy is, getting the scent of an essential oil to infuse itself into the atmosphere to create a pleasing and relaxing state of body and mind. To others is may be perceived as a relaxing massage session with the use of beneficial essential oils.

Using aromatherapy as a skin care regimen is also very popular. Many of the essential oils used have proven qualities that can contribute to the various needs addressed in skin care lines.

These requirements can range from wanting to keep the skin looking young and supple to actually reversing the aging effects on the skin. Some forms of eczema and acne have been successfully arrested with the use of the aromatherapy method.

Aromatherapy is also an excellent way recommended to get oneself into a meditative state. These meditative states are usually associated with yoga, tai chi, visualization or self hypnosis.

Trying various oils before deciding on the one that best allows you to reach the required level of mediation is sometimes needed. Besides this some research has shown that using aromatherapy can help create the mood for various scenarios with specific results in mind.

Though there is lack of conclusive evidence to show aromatherapy can be instrumental in treating certain diseases, the fact remains that many people turn to this alternative based on other success stories.

Traditionally linked to the successful treatment of emotional and physical ailments there is proven success because aromatherapy is a natural method that helps the body cope with stress, anxiety and tension which are all contributing factors or causes of other illnesses and diseases.

Chapter 6- Aromatherapy More than Just for Beauty

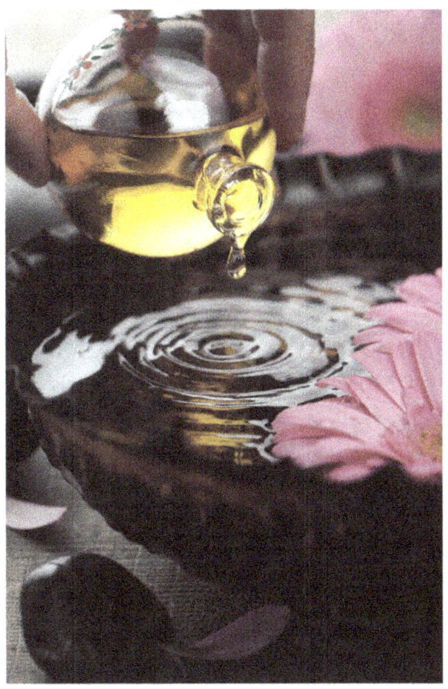

Aromatherapy has become very popular today. Though it is still mostly linked to idea of a relaxingly therapeutic massage session, newer uses are now being explored.

In ancient times aromatherapy was used for almost everything from relaxing to health solutions and even for culinary preparations. A lot needs to be understood before embarking on the journey of aromatherapy.

If one is thinking of setting up an aromatherapy centre or even considering the use of aromatherapy to treat a certain medical condition, the buying of the essential oils is a crucial aspect to consider.

Most essential oils today are so commercialized that it may not always be as genuine as stated on the labels. Careful examination of the label contents needs to be checked and rechecked before a purchase is made.

Some labels can be quite deceiving in their purported capabilities. The condition and type of packing of the essential oils is also a very important feature that should be considered. Ideally there should not be any cracks or broken seals as this will contribute to the contamination of the purity levels of the oils.

Besides all this, the other important fact to consider is getting the best results through the method and choice of essential oils. Meaning some essential oil work better when used the correct way and the best results are assured if the recommended way is not taken for granted but adhered to carefully.

The method of inhalation is used to treat certain ailments like sinuses, headaches, colds, chest congestions and other similar conditions. This method is far more effective and quicker than taking oral or direct application on the skin.

Spraying a mixture of essential oils and distilled water is another method used to create a calming and relaxing atmosphere. This method has proved to be beneficial when treating anxiety, depression, stress and other pressurizing conditions.

Some conditions call for direct applications. However as most aromatherapy massage session are performed with direct skin contact, the concentration of the essential oils needs to be considered before commencing. Reason being that these essential oils could cause an allergic reaction to the individual.

Commonly thought of as essential oils just for relaxing, therapeutic massage sessions, aromatherapy is fast gaining inroads into other areas. Some of which are forays into treating ailments and some medical conditions that have previous success rates from using aromatherapy methods.

What You Can Do

For years some cultures have used aromatherapy to treat wound and scars effectively. Using essential oils that contain the Helichrysum ingredient has been proven to be beneficial when repairing damaged skin conditions.

Its strong anti-inflammatory and concentration of regenerative diketones is what makes it a highly regarded compound in addressing damaged skin problems. The pleasing earthy aroma it emits is also therapeutic.

Other essential oils that are also known for their healing properties for skin conditions are lavender, sage and rosemary. Sage is particularly effective in healing old scars and stretch marks but should only be used is small amounts because of the Thujone content which can be toxic.

Using aromatherapy to treat wounds is also widely practiced. This is because of the antiseptic elements that certain essential oils contain. Tea tree essential oil is commonly used to treat wound until the wound is totally sealed, after which this oil is no longer needed.

Some aromatherapy treatments are also used when the desire for healthy, younger looking skin is sought. These essential oils are absorbed into the skin and in turn provide the skin with all the important nutrients needed for the healthy look and condition.

Aromatherapy is also used in other products besides skin care. Products such as bath salts, shower gels, shampoos, body lotions. This style of using aromatherapy is wonderful for creating the desired effects of sweet smelling and relaxing moods. Also aromatherapy in this form is mild and none threatening as it is not in its purest form.

Aromatherapy can also assist in relieving impatience and irritability. Essential oils like lavender can have calming effects on the mental turmoil state and works by encouraging the senses to slow down and simulates peace.

CHAPTER 7- AROMATHERAPY AND YOUR OVERALL WELLNESS

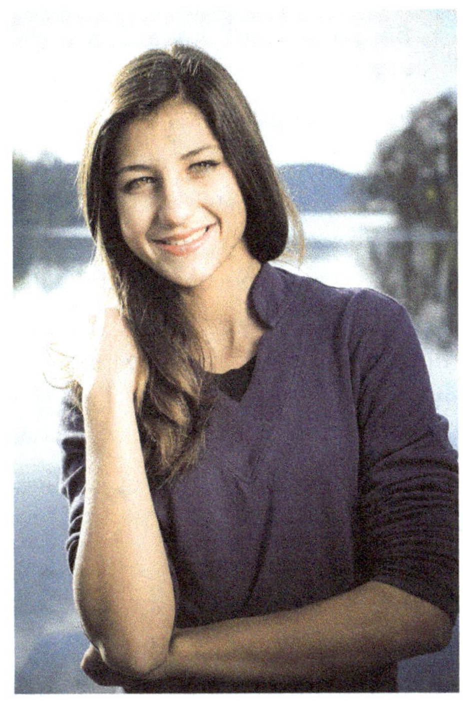

Approaching a medical condition by exploring the possibility of using aromatherapy as a solution is definitely worth the effort.

Aromatherapy ideally works when the psychological and physical aspects are addressed together. When the psychological and physical aspects are taken into account various contributing factors are studied carefully before any treatments are recommended.

The aroma therapist would have to consider factors like an individual's medical history, emotional condition, general health and lifestyle before putting forth any recommendations. This is a holistic style approach to treating a medical condition.

Some of the other more interesting conditions that are successfully explored using the aromatherapy method are backaches, irritable bowel syndrome, headaches and depression, to name a few. A good percentage of these medical ailments can be due to stress.

Thus by using methods to understand and locate the individual's stress causing source, the aroma therapist will be able to alleviate the medical condition in a more efficient manner. In some extreme cases, claims of total recovery have been documented.

Treating skin problems is another avenue where aromatherapy has been successfully used. Conditions such as dermatitis, acne, eczema, psoriasis, cellulite, varicose veins and stretch marks are just some of the conditions where the use of essential oils has either arrested the condition or eradicated it completely.

Some patients have used aromatherapy to combat depression, hysteria, lack of concentration and panic attacks. Having tried other medically accepted methods which sometimes have undesirable side effects, aromatherapy has become a welcome solution.

Treating burns, bruises and sprains using aromatherapy essential oils to achieve surprisingly quick and effective results are also another option worth exploring.

Other areas where the use of aromatherapy is being successfully explored are asthma, bronchitis, flu, and muscular aches and pains. When making the choice to use aromatherapy as a possible treatment for any given condition, it is important to ensure that only a qualified aromatherapy practitioner is consulted and that all the essential oils used are of the highest quality.

The popular belief that most illnesses and diseases are somehow linked to stress, anxiety and lack of proper daily nutrition has its merits.

Unfortunately some illnesses and diseases need to reach a critical stage before it becomes visible or is detected. To avoid all this, one is encouraged, though unrealistically, to keep all negative aspects in life under control or eliminate them altogether.

Wellness

Aromatherapy can helpfully contribute to this end. Primarily known for its calming properties, aromatherapy methods advocate the use of various essential oils to soothe the mind and body. Besides this a long list of other conditions can be successfully addressed with the use of aromatherapy elements.

Below are just a few examples of the capabilities and merits of using aromatherapy:

• Acne – lavender oil or tea tree oil to be applied directly onto the affected area. For milder cases, using a body bath lotion with these properties is recommended.

• Anemia – a concoction of tincture from the yellow dock root or an extract of dandelion leaf or even eating dandelion greens as a salad.

• Anxiety – chamomile, California poppy, passion flower, lemon balm

• Asthma – ginkgo biloba, mullein oil, a Chinese herb called shuan huang lian

• Bee sting – urtica urens, cantharis, lavender and vegetable oil mixed

• Body odor – alfalfa contains chlorophyll.

• Cold – eucalyptus oil in boiling water and inhaled. Gargle with a mixture of tea tree oil

• Cholesterol – chicory root, ginger

• Constipation – aloe vera juice, ginger tea

• Hair loss – saw palmetto, arnica, jojoba oil

• Headaches – chamomile relaxes, ginkgo biloba improves blood circulation

• Dandruff – flaxseed oil, primrose oil or salmon oil. Rinsing hair in chaparral or thyme

• Diabetes – huckleberry, tea made from most beans

• Diarrhea – blackberry tea, wild oregano

• Eczema – chickweed added to bath, stinging nettle, hazel ointment

• Indigestion – gentian root for better digestion, ginger, peppermint

• Nausea and vomiting – catnip leaves, chamomile flowers

• Menopause – for skin use geranium essential oil, orange blossom water, sandalwood essential oil

Aromatherapy and Healing

Fast gaining popularity as a new age fad, aromatherapy is only recently being taken seriously as a viable alternative treatment method to conventional medical remedies. For most ancient cultures this method of treatment has long been practiced with successful results.

More In Depth Healing Info

Confusing the attributes that come with using the term aromatherapy is mainly caused by the commercial sector seeking to capitalize in this area. For many people aromatherapy is usually linked to some pleasing scent emitted from essential oils.

The effectiveness in the aromatherapy element is in the application and intent. Aromatherapy is meant to create a positive change physically, emotionally, mentally or spiritually which is supposed to directly impact the body condition of the person undergoing a session.

However when products are touted to use or contain essential oils for aromatherapy purposes without actually comprising of the much needed dosage, it is no longer considered aromatherapy.

Aromatherapy or commonly referred to as the practice of using essential oils for medicinal and therapeutic purposes covers many areas of healing properties. There are many essential oils used as remedies for various physical conditions and complaints. Essential oils are also believed to contain anti-viral, anti-fungal and anti-bacterial properties. There are also some essential oils that work well for various skin problems.

CHAPTER 8- TIPS ON HOW TO PROPERLY USE AROMATHERAPY

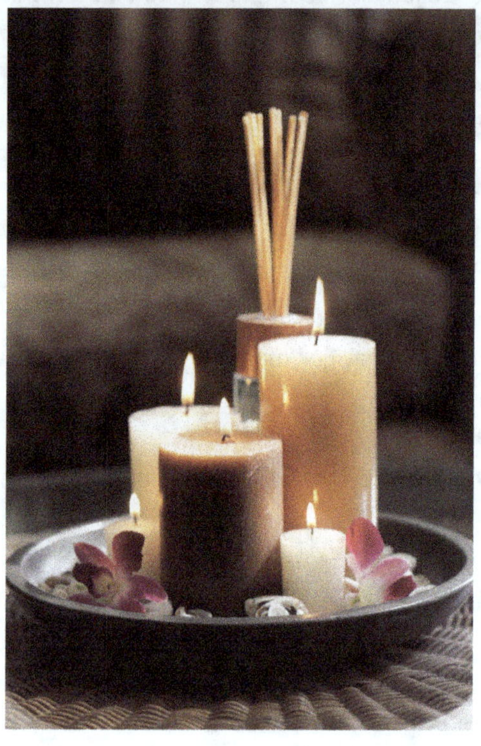

The term aromatherapy has been so loosely used over the years for commercial reasons that it has become almost totally misleading.

Understood to mean a combination of two basic words – aroma and therapy, the word aromatherapy has been commercially used so widely that many false claims have been made over the years to promote and capitalize on it. A little time and research should shed light on this confusion.

Aromatherapy is actually a serious foray to embark upon as it involves the use of pure essential oil and other natural ingredients that are considered safe to use only if done correctly. Not understanding the attributes and purity of aromatherapy, can lead serious repercussion as not all natural and pure oils are safe for human use. Some essential oils can even be toxic in certain circumstances.

Pregnant women and lactating mothers should be weary when choosing to use aromatherapy. The strong scents can be harmful to babies as their senses and immune system are not fully developed yet. Also some scents can be off putting to the baby and this may affect the baby's sleep patterns and feeding schedules, thus causing health issues from the neo natal stage.

Though aromatherapy has calming effects, using some essential oils to sooth and relax a cancer patient may have adverse effects. A doctor's permission should always be sought before trying this form of therapy. Some of the essential oils may have negative reactions to the prescription drugs already taken by the patient.

The choice made to use aromatherapy as an alternative to other medical options, should only be done after extensive studies have been made on the advantages and disadvantages.

Although most illnesses and diseases are found to be the root cause of stress, anxiety and other pressurizing conditions, opting to treat the medical condition by using aromatherapy may produce minimal positive results to actually combating the disease or illness.

Overenthusiastic use or indulgence of aromatherapy can lead to serious problems, especially when medical advice has been ignored in making this choice. Some studies continually show little of no evidence in demonstrating efficacy against bacterial, fungal or viral infections, thus rendering it a poor alternative to medically proven alternatives.

In most countries around the world, the aromatherapy use is still related to the indulgent relaxing aspect. Hence there is no regulatory body that strictly governs the content and potency of each essential oil used for the aromatherapy session.

Undiluted essential oils used for aromatherapy can sometime cause skin irritations and discolorations. In cases where the natural product has been exposed to chemicals in their growing stage, such as pesticides, chemical allergies can have a negative effect upon application. In more severe cases the presence of estrogens like elements, have been found to negatively affect the delicate skin of children.

Some cultures take the aromatherapy influence to the extreme. Ingesting certain ingredients is widely practiced and sometimes causes severe irreparable damage. As some of the essential can be quite toxic when ingested, medical advice should always be sought before advocating such a choice.

As with any bioactive substances the method of aromatherapy, using essential oils, and while safe for the general public can still have adverse effects when used by pregnant or lactating women.

Some of the ingredients and methods used in a particular aromatherapy session may cause negative side effects when interaction with other more conventional medicinal elements are present. Adulterated oils used in some aromatherapy sessions can also pose problems depending on the type of substance used.

Other safety issue like the unsubstantiated claims made by those advocating aromatherapy as a proven alternative treatment can be misleading at best.

What's Good and What's Not

Aromatherapy and essential oils are linked, and so when considering using this method for treatments or for other reasons, taking the time and effort to understand the fundamentals of aromatherapy is essential.

Essential because limited knowledge of aromatherapy can cause the wrong use of the essential oils, wrong methods of applications chosen or even the use of products which actually don't contain any essential oils at all.

Poor quality oils severely lack the optimum benefits it promotes itself to have. In the course of processing these oils many factors should be considered if the end product is to provide what it promises to. Some of the things to consider are; if there are added chemicals, preservatives, substandard quality of ingredients, poor processing environments and adulteration of the oils. All these factors are important because harmful side effects can occur if other than the required essential oil is contained in the packaging. At best only minimal therapeutic benefits can be derived.

Some vendors combine the essential oils with other chemical and lesser grade ingredients for higher profit gains. These oils then become either useless or less effective. Label words like fragrance oil, natural identical oil, and perfume oil are all words that are misleading in nature. As there are no strict guide lines to follow, some vendors intentionally or unintentionally use words like therapeutic grade or aromatherapy grade, thus these terms should be ignored and the contents examined closely.

Packaging styles are also another important factor to consider. Don't be misled by pretty packaging as it is the content that is important. Also essential oils that are packaged in darker colored bottle can be the way a vendor "hides" the clarity and purity of its content. The use of plastic style packaging is also not wise as some essential oils react with the plastic, thus causing the quality of the said oil to deteriorate considerably.

Chapter 9- Tips on How to Make Money with Aromatherapy

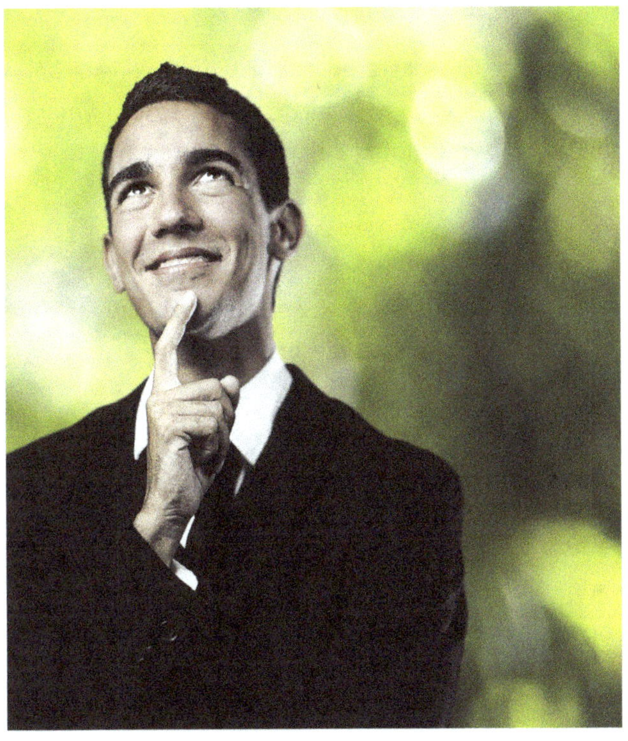

Now that you have learned so much about this miraculous healing remedy of aromatherapy and what it can do, you can choose to incorporate it into your everyday life. Be forewarned, however, that aromatherapy is addictive. Once you start making bath salts and massage oils, you will want to make more and more things.

The list of what you can make when it come to aromatherapy is long. In addition to what we described throughout the book, other items you can make to incorporate aromatherapy include shampoos, soaps, moisturizers, lotions and potpourri. The possibilities are endless. You may decide to start making "healing baskets" for friends and relatives. You can purchase some pretty bottles and containers and decorate them with ribbons. The choices are endless.

Once you have really mastered the art of making aromatherapy products at home, you may want to begin to sell your products. Before you do this, you should be aware of one caveat:

We live in a very litigious society. Be careful whenever you sell any sort of healing product to people because they are likely to sue if something goes wrong.

In order to continue your business without worrying about getting sued by some money hungry lawyer, you should do the following before you sell a thing that has to do with aromatherapy:

⚕   Add a disclaimer to the product stating that it is not for medical use;

⚕   Incorporate your business

A disclaimer will let people know that you are not making any sort of medical claims about the product. You have to be very careful about selling   healing products   h on the market today because people will be very quick to file a lawsuit if it doesn't   ft work. You cannot go about saying that you can cure someone with terminal cancer with lavender - it is not only wrong, but you are giving the family false hope.

That being said, there are cases where people who were written off as hopeless   h   by   doctors,   have   bounced   back   using aromatherapy or

other alternative therapies. We have to get out of the mindset that doctors are not God. They have a lot of the answers, but not all. And every once in a while, something happens that stumps them. Where there is life, there is hope.

You should be cautioned, however, about preying on people who are seriously ill and promising them cures. This is not only inaccurate and unproven, but it is bad karma. Don ft do it. Promote your product as a way to treat minor. After all, if pharmaceutical companies can sell gold medicine h over the counter, you can also sell aromatherapy products. The only difference is that your stuff will actually work and won ft have any side effects.

Put a legal disclaimer on all of your products and literature that this is made for the following:

External use only. Keep away from eyes. Keep away from children. Not meant to be a substitute for medical treatment. Do not use on sensitive skin. Do not use on broken skin areas. Do not use in mouth or genital area.

The other thing you should do is incorporate. Not all businesses need to incorporate, but those who sell items such as aromatherapy healing products are wise to incorporate their business. This can protect your personal assets.

A corporation is like a separate entity. It can open bank accounts, file taxes and be sued. The owner of the corporation is the stockholders. The names of the stockholders are not public record; the names of the officers running the company are public record. In most small businesses, the stockholders and the officers are the same people.

It is not difficult to open a corporation. You need a tax number from the federal government called an FEIN and you need to file Articles of Incorporation with the state. The fee to file Articles of Incorporation varies from state to state. It is usually around $100.

The form is simple to fill out and there are various places online that can do this for you cheaply. Although corporations are required to hold annual meetings of stockholders and officers as well as have a corporate resolution whenever a decision is made, if you are the only one in the corporation, you can do this any time you want. It can be written on a piece of paper. Save yourself the money and skip the "corporate book and seal" deal.

You don't need it in a small corporation that is not offering public stocks. In fact, you don't really need to do anything except pay your taxes and file an annual report, which you will get from the state and, essentially, gets mailed back signed stating that nothing has changed.

For a small fee, you can protect yourself against any sue happy lawyer that wants to sue you for selling their client massage oil that made them break out for a few days and caused them mental distress. h

Aromatherapy products can be a big business and quite profitable. You just want to be sure that you protect your own personal assets. If you selling your products under the corporation, they cannot go after you personally for anything.

Where To Sell Your Aromatherapy Products

Many of us who use the internet for business purposes still find it amazing that some businesses do not have a website. If you decide to get into the aromatherapy business, make sure that you develop a professional looking website. One way to draw people to your website is through content. Continue to post articles on your site about the benefits of aromatherapy to make sure your site comes up in the search engines.

Do not limit your selling only to your online website. Craft fairs are an excellent place to sell your products. There are craft fairs in every town throughout the year. Some people actually make their living selling products by traveling to craft fairs all year long.

Craft fairs are actually better than the internet when it comes to selling aromatherapy. Make sure that you set up your booth to appear pleasant and tranquil and have some incense burning. Put some products out for samples and make sure they are displayed pleasantly. Use wrappings such as ribbons, nice bottles and tissue paper. If you can, get labels with a logo and name and number on it of your corporation so that customer can place re-orders.

Decorative packaging is key to selling aromatherapy products. People will not only want them for themselves, but for gifts for other people. You can actually have quite a lucrative business by selling aromatherapy products.

Another place you can sell your products are independent beauty salons. While salons that have full service spas will have their own line of products they wish to sell, other salons do not. You can offer the salon a commission if they allow you to place your products in their store and if they sell.

Salons are not the only places where you can sell your products. Boutiques that are independently owned will want to carry your products if they look professional. Make sure that you have labels on the bottles and that soaps and other items are wrapped in proper papers with labels. The more professional the product appears the more money it can sell for and the better chance you have of it being accepted into an upscale boutique.

Offer healing gift baskets for people. Gift baskets are popular and can be a profitable business all on their own. Start an aromatherapy gift basket business and watch your business start to boom. Can you imagine a more appropriate gift for a person coming home from surgery or someone who just had a baby than a pretty basket packed with aromatherapy goodies?

You can not only enjoy aromatherapy in your home and with your family, but you can also make a profitable business as more people are beginning to discover the joys of aromatherapy.

Chapter 10- Quick Reference on Aromatherapy

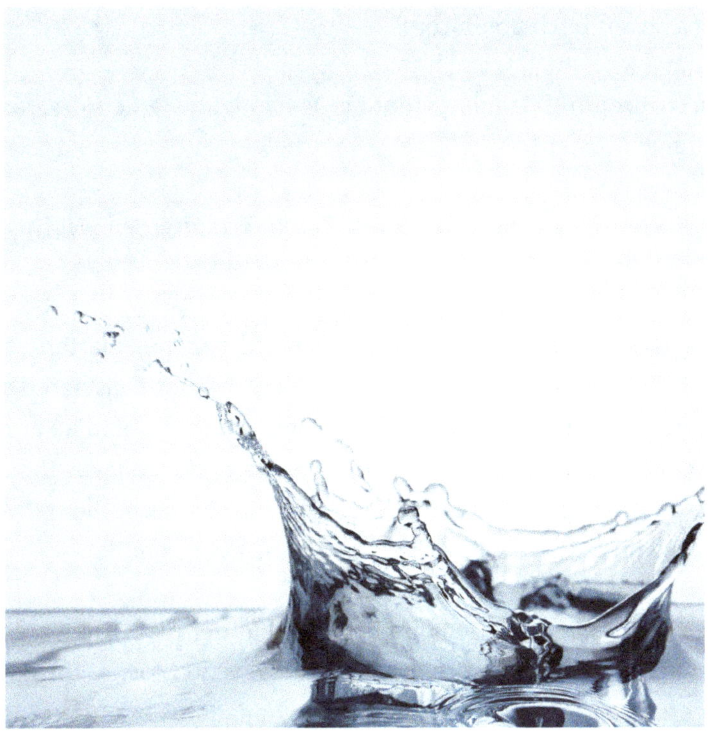

Dangerous Essential Oils

The following is a list of essential oils that should never be used by an amateur. This is a warning in case you purchase oils from a disreputable dealer overseas who may not be aware of the toxicity of these oils.

Chances are that you will never come across them, but you should still be well aware of the dangerous essential oils that should not be used in aromatherapy:

Ajowan

Bitter Almond

Arnica Sweet Birch Boldo Leaf

Spanish Broom Calamus Camphor Deertongue Garlic Horseradish Jaborandi Mustard

Onion Pennyroyal Rue Sassafras Thuja Wintergreen Wormseed Wormwood

While these essential oils have their place in other matters, they should not be used in aromatherapy. They are not considered safe to breath in. Funny enough that camphor, once a use in all homes for colds, is among the group. However, camphor today is thought to promote respiratory problems instead of cure them. Most people who grew up with this remedy, however, lived.

While garlic and onion may be beneficial in our diets, they are not recommended for their scent. We all know that. Most of the above dangerous essential oils are considered dangerous because of their strong odor and irritant qualities. Chances are that you will not be seeing any of these oils in any of the places you purchase your essential oils.

A Guide To 60 Popular Essential Oils And Their Uses

1. Angelica Root. This has a spicy and woodsy scent and is used as a base note in perfumery. It can be used to treat skin conditions but should be avoided during pregnancy. It is also phototoxic.

2. Anise. This is a popular plant that tastes and smells like licorice. It

is very sweet and is a top note in perfumery. It can be used for colds, aches and flatulence. It should not be used in women who have a history of breast or ovarian cancer or endometriosis.

3. Peru Balsam. A sweet scent and very woodsy. It is used as a base note in perfumes and can be used in aromatherapy for rashes, stress, chapped skin or the flu.

4. Basil. A sweet scent that has a reek of camphor and is a top note in perfume. A popular herb for cooking, basil essential oil can be used to treat colds coughs flatulence and even as an insect repellent. High doses of basil, however, can be hazardous.

5. Bay. Bay has a spicy aroma and is a middle note when used in perfumes. It can be used for dandruff, oily skin and sprains. In the case of someone with kidney or liver problems, or who is taking anticoagulants, it should be avoided. Those who have a history of prostate cancer or alcoholism should also avoid using bay.

6. Bay Laurel. Bay Laurel has a fruity scent and is a top note in perfumes. It can be used to treat colds or flue and even tonsillitis. It should not be used in pregnancy.

7. Beeswax. Beeswax has a very sweet scent and is used as a base note in perfumery. It has no therapeutic value but is valued for its pleasant scent in perfumery.

8. Benzoin. Benzoin has a woodsy aroma that is very rich and is used as a base note in perfumery. It can be used for arthritis, chapped skin and stress. It is relatively safe to use but persons who use it should check for skin allergies.

9. Bergamot. This has a very citrus like scent and is a top note in perfumery. It is used to treat acne, cold sores, psoriasis, stress and

boils. It is photo toxic so if you use bergamot, avoid the sun for twelve hours after treatment.

10. Bergamot Mint. Like bergamot, it has a citrus like scent and is minty. It is also a top note in perfumery and is used to treat cramps and upset stomach.

11. Rosewood. It has a sweet yet woodsy and floral fragrance that is an excellent middle note in perfumes. It is used to treat acne, colds, headaches and other minor skin conditions.

12. Boronia. Boronia has a very floral scent and is mostly used in perfumery as a strong top note.

13. Cajeput. Cajeput has a camphor like aroma but is slightly fruity. It is a middle note in perfumery and is used to treat colds, coughs, aches and sore throat.

14. Cardamum. Cardamum has a spicy and woodsy scent and is a middle note in perfumery. It is used to treat fatigue and stress.

15. Carrot Seed. Carrot Seed has a woodsy scent and is a medium note in perfumery. It is used to treat wrinkles, eczema and gout.

16. Atlas Cedarwood. There are different types of cedar wood - Atlas and Virginia. Atlas cedarwood has a woodsy scent that is used as a medium note in perfumery. It is used to treat coughing, stress, dermatitis, acne and arthritis. It should be avoided during pregnancy.

17. Virginia Cedarwood. This has a scent that is what you smell in cedar chests. Very woodsy and a medium note in perfumery. It has the same medicinal uses as Atlas Cedarwood but is also used as an

insect repellent. This may be safer to use than Atlas Cedarwood but should not be used by pregnant women.

18. German Chamomile. There are two different types of Chamomile - German and Roman. German Chamomile is sweet and used as a medium note in perfumery. It has many uses including the treatment of minor skin conditions, earaches, headache, nausea, PMS, stress, arthritis, sprains and stress. It is relatively very safe to use but should be checked for skin reactions

19. Roman Chamomile. Pretty much like German Chamomile and is also a medium but stronger note in perfumery. There is little difference between German and Roman Chamomile.

20. Cinnamon. Cinnamon has a spicy scent and is strong middle note in perfumery. It can be used to treat constipation, low blood pressure, lice and stress. It should be avoided in people who have a history of liver or kidney problems or prostrate cancer. It should also be avoided by anyone taking anticoagulants or has a history of alcoholism.

21. Citronella. It has a citrus like scent that is used as a top note in perfumery. It makes an excellent insect repellent and is often used in candles in this manner. It can also treat fatigue, oily skin and headaches.

22. Clary Sage. Clary Sage has an slightly sweet aroma and is a middle note in perfumery. It is used to treat gas, sore throats, coughing, exhaustion and stress.

23. Clove Bud. Spicy and woodsy it is a strong middle note in perfumery. It is used to treat arthritis, toothaches and sprains as well as rheumatism. Is should be avoided in people with kidney,

liver or prostrate problems or who have a history of alcohol abuse. Those taking anticoagulants should also not take this healing oil.

24. Coriander. Coriander is a spicy and woodsy essential oil that has a nice middle note for perfumery. It is used to treat aches and pains, indigestion, nausea and fatigue.

25. Cypress. Cypress has a woodsy scent that reminds you of evergreen trees. It is a middle note in perfumery and is used to treat perspiration, hemorrhoids, oily skin and rheumatism.

26. Dill. Dill has a sweet scent and is used as a middle note in perfumery. It is used to treat aches and pains as well as flatulence.

27. Elemi. This has a spicy yet citrus like scent and is a middle note in perfumery. It is used to treat coughing as well as wrinkles and stress. It can also be used to put on wounds. Use sparingly and with caution as research as to the effects of this essential oil have not yet been completed.

28. Eucalyptus. This has a top note in perfumery as it is very woodsy and fresh. It is used to treat cold sores, colds, coughing, flue and sinusitis. It can be very toxic if taken internally and is strictly for external use only.

29. Lemon Eucalyptus. Similar to the uses of Eucalyptus but with a lemony scent and a use as a middle note in perfumery. It can be safer to use than regular Eucalyptus.

30. Radiata Eucalyptus. This has a sweet scent and is used as a middle note in perfumery. It is also used for relatively the same treatments as lemon and regular Eucalyptus.

31. Fennel. Fennel has a licorice like scent to it and is used as both a top and medium note in perfumery. It can be used to treat flatulence, nausea, bad breath, obesity and water retention. It should be avoided with people who have a history of breast or ovarian cancer, hyperplasia, endometriosis or prostate cancer.

32. Fir Needle. This has a woodsy scent and is used as a middle note in perfumery. It is used to treat colds, coughs, flu, rheumatism and general aches and pains.

33. Frankincense. Spicy, woodsy and fruity, Frankincense is a base note in perfumery. It can be used to treat anxiety, stress, coughing and even for scars and stretch marks.

34. Galbanum. A woodsy and spicy scent that is used as a top note in perfumery, Galbanum is used to treat skin irritations, acne, lice, wrinkles and muscle aches.

35. Geranium. There are two different types of Geranium - regular Geranium and Rose Geranium. Geranium has a sweet scent that is used to as a middle note in perfumery. It is used to treat acne and oily skin and also as a relief for symptoms of menopause. It should be avoided during pregnancy.

36. Rose Geranium. Rose Geranium is used for primarily the same purposes as regular geranium but has a more floral scent. It is also used as a middle note in perfumery.

37. Ginger. Ginger has a very spicy and woodsy scent and is used as both a middle and base note in perfumery. Ginger is used to treat nausea as well as aching muscles and arthritis. It can be phototoxic so avoid the sun for 12 hours after use.

38. Grapefruit. Very citrus like scent and is used as a top note in perfumery. It can treat dull skin and water retention. It should not be used in the sunlight as it can be photo toxic. Avoid the sun 12 hours after using Grapefruit essential oils.

39. Helichyrsum. A spicy base note in perfumery it is used to treat minor skin conditions, particularly wounds.

40. Hyssop. A fruity yet woodsy scent, it is a middle note in perfumery and is used to treat coughing and sore throat. It should be avoided by anyone with epilepsy or with a fever. It should not be used if you are pregnant or on children.

41. Immortelle. A spicy base note used in perfumery, it is used to treat minor skin conditions, including acne and burns, cuts and irritated skin.

42. Jasmine. A floral and Oriental scent, it is used as a Middle note in perfumery. It is used to treat depression, stress, dry skin and even labor pains. It has also been used as an aphrodisiac.

43. Juniper Berry. This has a sweet and almost fruity scent and is used as a middle note in perfumery. It is used to treat cellulites, gout, hemorrhoids and also rheumatism. It should not be used by pregnant women or in people with liver problems.

44. Lavender. Lavender has a floral scent and is used as a top note in perfumery. It is used to treat just about everything - from acne to vertigo. It is one of the safest of all of the essential oils and one of the few that can be used directly on the skin. Lavender buds are also boiled like tea and consumed internally.

45. Lemon. Citrus scent like lemons only much stronger in an essential oil. It is used as a top note in perfumery and is also used

to treat athlete's foot, colds, oily skin, acne, and even warts. Like most of the citrus derived essential oils, it is photo toxic and should not be used in the sunlight.

46. Lemongrass. Has a lemony scent that is also used as a top note in perfume. The medicinal purposes of this essential oil are similar to lemon, but it can also be used to treat flatulence and as an insect repellant. It should not be used on children or with people who have an enlarged prostrate or glaucoma.

47. Lime. A citrus scent used as a top note in perfumes and treats the same things as lemon essential oil. As with lemon and grapefruit and other citrus essential oils, it is photo toxic so avoid the sunlight 12 hours after using lime essential oil.

48. Mandarin. Has a citrus scent and is used as a top note in perfumery. It is good for wrinkles and minor skin conditions. It has also been known to treat insomnia.

49. Myrrh. Myrrh has a woodsy scent and is used as a base note in perfumery. It is used to treat bad breath, hemorrhoids, minor rashes and toothaches among other things. It should never be taken internally.

500. Neroli. Both floral and citrus, this is used as a middle note in a perfumery base and acts as a treatment for mild depression, insomnia and is a potent aphrodisiac.

51. Nutmeg. A rich and spicy scent that is used as a middle note in perfumery. Nutmeg is also used to treat constipation, fatigue, nausea and aches and pains. It can be toxic if used in large amount. If taken orally to an extreme, can produce effects similar to hallucinogenic drugs.

52. Orange. There are two types of orange - bitter and sweet. Both are top notes in perfumery and sweet orange, as its name implies, is sweeter. Both are used to treat constipation, colds, flatulence, and stress. Sunlight should be avoided for 12 hours after using orange essential oil.

53. Patchouli. A woodsy scent that is used as a base note in perfumery. It is used to treat acne, minor skin conditions, stress and as an insect repellent. It is also a powerful aphrodisiac.

54. Peppermint. It has a minty scent and is used as a top note in perfumery. It is used to treat headache, nausea and flatulence as well as vertigo. It should not be used if a person has a fever and should not be taken internally as it can be toxic. Those with epilepsy should avoid taking peppermint.

55. Rose. Rose has as a floral scent and is used as a middle note in perfumery. It is used to treat stress, depression and symptoms of menopause. It is also used as somewhat of an aphrodisiac. Rose is one of the safest of all of the essential oils.

56. Sandalwood. Used as a base note in perfumery, the scent is both woodsy and floral and very rich. It can be used to treat mild depression and skin conditions.

57. Spearmint. It has a minty scent and is used as a top note in perfumery. It is used to treat basically the same minor ailments as peppermint.

58. Tea Tree. There are three types of Tea Tree - Common, Lemon and New Zealand. Both Common and New Zealand Tea Tree have a middle perfumery note and a woodsy scent. Lemon Tea Tree has a top note and a sweeter scent. Uses for all Tea Tree include acne,

stress, cold sores, colds, flu, insect bites, migraine headaches, oily skin, warts and athlete's foot.

59. Vanilla. Vanilla has a strong, sweet scent that is used as a base note in perfumery. It is one of the few essential oils that is safe to use directly on the skin. Vanilla can be used as a stress reliever, but it is mostly used in perfumery.

60. Ylang Ylang. A sweet and floral fragrance that is used as a base and middle note in perfumery. Ylang Ylang is used to treat anxiety, mild depression, stress and is a powerful aphrodisiac.

Note that the conditions listed above are mild conditions. Those who have severe medical conditions are urged not to attempt to treat themselves but visit a physician.

Essential oils should not be used directly on the skin, with the exception of lavender and vanilla.

Essential oils should not be taken internally - they are for external use only. Lavender and chamomile are often dried and sold as teas; however, the essential oils should not be taken orally.

Aromatherapy oils are safe when used as directed. If you have a condition that is not clearing up after treatment with aromatherapy, or if the problem is getting worse, see you doctor.

About the Author

Helga Shaffer is very passionate on what she is doing and one of the best. Helga is internationally known as an aromatherapist and a certified holistic instructor. Helga promotes the natural way of taking care of our well-being rather than relying on chemical based treatment.

Due to her long list of experience and expertise when it comes to aromatherapy, Helga has taught seminars in different associations and institutions, mainly in California. She is also often invited to give lecture on the said topic.

www.ingramcontent.com/pod-product-compliance
Lightning Source LLC
Chambersburg PA
CBHW050656250726

48662CB00002B/708